Organic Fitness

GOD'S EXERCISE MANUAL

10 EXERCISES TO PERFECT HEALTH

BUILD AN EMPIRE

1. FOUNDATIONAL SQUAT

2. FOUNDATIONAL PUSHUP

3. YOGA SQUAT

4. YOGA PUSHUP

5. PLEA SQUAT

6. ELBOWS IN PUSHUP

7. ABDOMINAL CRUNCH

8. REVERSE CRUNCH

9. TRANSVERSE CRUNCH

10. BACK EXTENSION

Table of Contents

Foreword

These are God's exercises because they are God's movements. Sitting and standing, pushing yourself up from the ground, and getting up from the ground are all essential to life. The ability to perform these movements is the ability and freedom to live. Do not be a prisoner in your own body be free to run, jump, play, and love. These are simple and easy exercises but must be practiced to perfection, until your body is perfect like God intended, making you an image of God.

The exercises in the book are intended for everyone. The exercises in this book can heal an injury, and they can make anyone healthier. With the 10 exercises featured in this book, anyone can lose weight if he or she is overweight. The exercises are progressive. There is an alternative to every exercise. If you practice the exercises, progression is unavoidable. If an exercise is difficult, it will become less difficult. If an exercise is not possible for you to perform, it soon will be possible for you to perform it with perfect form. Every exercise is a progression in your fitness. Your body will lead you to a happier state of mind.

It is your thoughts that will provide your health. You must perceive activity as something that is good for you and something that you enjoy doing. There are times for being still and times for being active. You must dedicate a time for activity in your life. Time should not be a factor. You do not skip a day brushing your teeth, or showering, so you will not miss another day of activity take the time to make yourself look better and feel better. If you have only one minute for exercise, then you can perform 30 Yoga squats in that time there is no excuse to not be fit. If you have two minutes, you can accomplish 30 Yoga squats and 30 Yoga pushups. If you have three minutes, you can accomplish 30 Yoga squats, 30 Yoga pushups, and 30 plea squats, and that is quite a workout if done in perfect form.

To make any change in your body, changing your mind must be the first step. Exercise is 90% mental and 10% physical. You must make a commitment in your mind before you perform one repetition of one exercise. You must make the decision that exercise is going to help you. You have to make the decision for yourself that activity will make you feel better, look better, and be happier. One million doctors, lawyers, judges, and studies cannot decide for you. More than one million studies have been published, and more than one million educated people have documented that exercise will make you healthier, happier, look better, and feel better. YOU have to do it. And before you do it, you must have the thought and the feeling that it is good for you and you want to do it. If you fear or do not enjoy activity then it will not save your life. It will consume time in your life. Do yourself a favor and believe. Believe so much you can feel it. Feel it so much that you have to move. Move the way the next few chapters describe in detail. Follow every instruction perfectly, and repeat the exercises until they are perfect. Repeat every cue next to every picture over and over, until your body is illustrating perfect form. Then send me a picture! TheOrganicWorkout.com. There will be an estimation of repetitions completed per minute for each exercise. Try to follow this estimate for a challenging workout. You should try to not include a rest in your short workout. Dedicate at least five minutes towards your health every day. If you miss one day then double up, 10 minutes, the next day. Do 20 minutes of activity if you miss yet another day. No one's schedule is perfect, only you are. Exercise to perfection.

Never ignore pain; pain is an indication to stop.

Foundational Exercises

Steel Legs and Iron Shirt

The foundational exercises in this book can provide endless health benefits. Form is of absolute importance. If you do not perform proper form you will not yield the intended results. Without perfect form, you are not doing the intended exercise, and may hurt yourself. If an athlete can hurt himself or herself with a slight movement then it is more than likely an untrained person will damage himself or herself.

Intensity is just as important as the form. Without intensity, you cannot expect results. Intensity must be at the level your body requires adaptation. If your body is not challenged enough to "adapt" to your workout, you will not see change in your body or performance level. Lactic acid is your best judge of intensity. "Feel the burn!" Lactic acid is the slight burning sensation localized to the specific muscle group that is being trained.

You will burn more than 100 calories in just five minutes with a single exercise. You will increase your metabolism for hours with a single exercise. You will increase your metabolism permanently with a single exercise.

33 repetitions in a minute will make you healthier

FOUNDATIONAL SQUAT
STEEL LEGS

~FEET SLIGHTLY WIDER THAN SHOULDER WIDTH APART

~TOES POINTED SLIGHTLY OUT TO REDUCE TORQUE ON KNEE

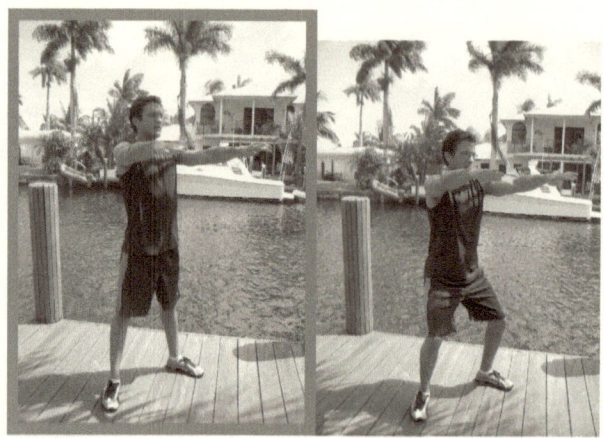

~Knees stabilized directly over ankles throughout entire motion

~Hands extended in front of body

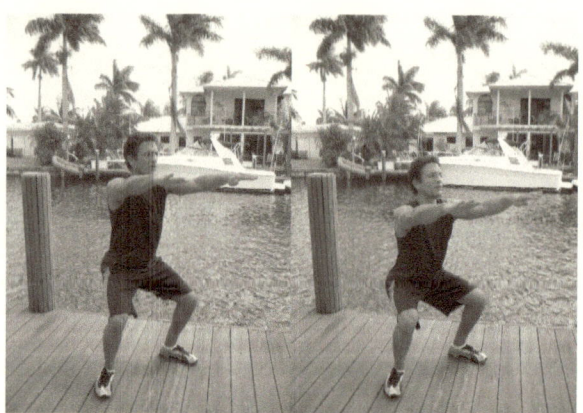

~Abdominals and lower back flexed and tight

~Muscles tightened throughout body as if absorbing impact

~Push the hips back as if sitting in a chair

~Do not push knees forward

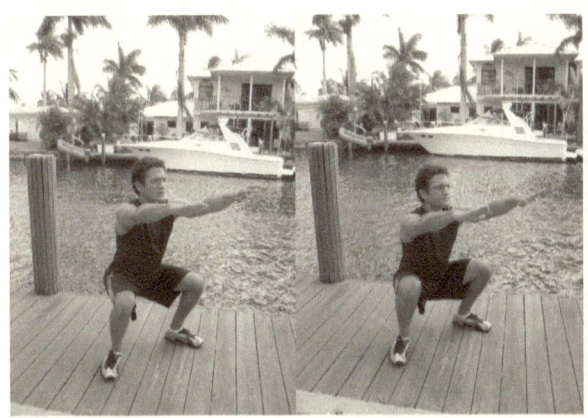

~FLEX LOWER BACK SO SHOULDERS ARE ALIGNED OVER HIPS

~FOCUS ALL YOUR WEIGHT ON YOUR HEELS, USING TOES ONLY TO STABILIZE

~SLOWLY LOWER BODYWEIGHT USING YOUR HAMSTRINGS

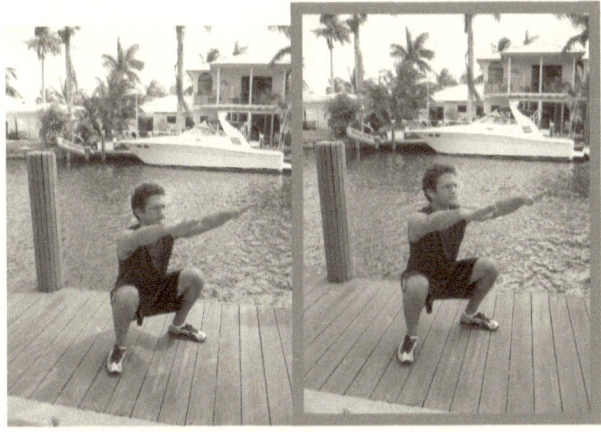

~PAUSE AND LIFT YOUR BODY SLOWLY WITH ABSOLUTE CONTROL

~SQUAT LOW WITH NO PAIN, HIPS BELOW KNEES TO CONTRACT GLUTES

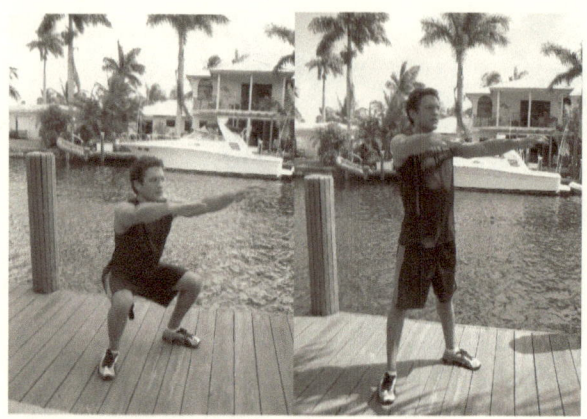

-Repeat until lactic acid slows your motion, with no pause at top

Foundational Squat
Steel Legs

In theory, your legs are your second heart. They are your number-one source of venous blood return. This means they bring blood back to your heart. Weakness in the legs is directly linked to complications in the hospital. Blood clots may appear due to bed rest and may cause an aneurism. Doing foundational squats will build capillaries, which will increase blood flow by creating new sources of blood flow through arteries and veins.

Doing this squat for just one minute will increase your metabolism. You must do the squat perfectly, as noted in the diagram above. You must flex your abdominals so that your shoulders are directly over your hips. Your spine must be absolutely straight as if it were a steel rod. Although you have a natural S curve in your spine, you must picture a steel rod through your spine to allow for perfect alignment.

Form is essential, and so is intensity. **Intensity will be monitored in two different methods:**

1.) Lactic acid, the burning in your muscle

2.) Anaerobic threshold, being out of breath (but able to speak)

In just one minute, you may achieve an anaerobic threshold. With one single exercise, you can reach this metabolic-enhancing threshold. Performing this one exercise to absolute perfection will get you in perfect shape. Being in good shape is reflected in every part of your life. Just one exercise, performed perfectly for just one minute, can and will make you healthier. It will make everything in life easier. In just one minute, out of the 1,440 minutes you have in a day, you can obtain a healthier body and a more focused mind.

50 repetitions in a minute will make you healthier

FOUNDATIONAL PUSHUP
IRON SHIRT

~PLANK POSITION WITH WRISTS ALIGNED UNDER SHOULDERS

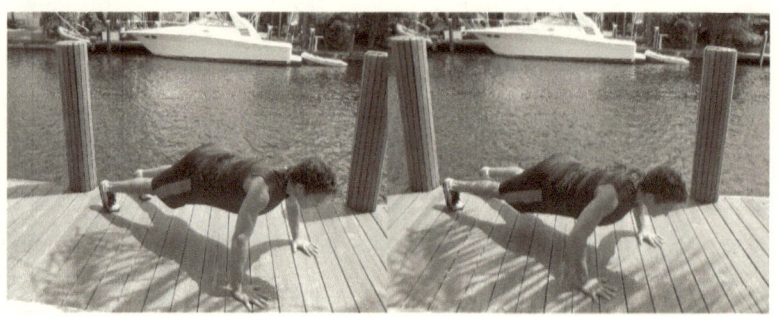

~WEIGHT FOCUSED ON THE PALMS OF THE HANDS, FINGERS STABILIZED

~Abdominals, buttocks, and muscles surrounding armpits TIGHT

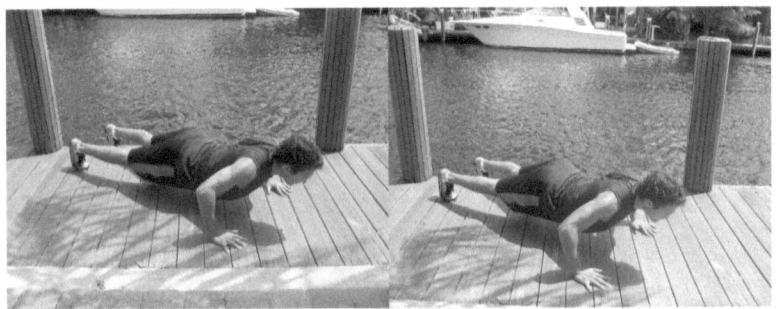

~The spine is imagined as a steel rod, preventing risk of injury

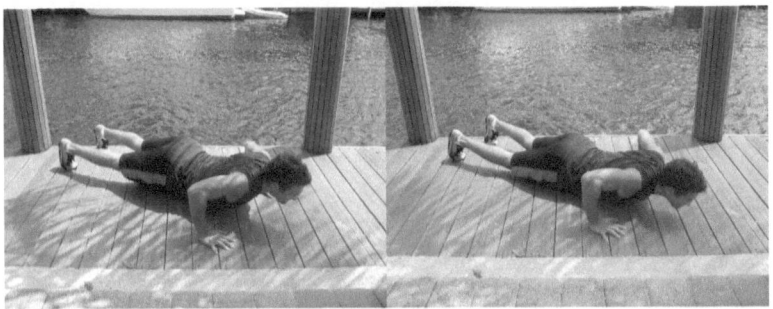

~Muscles tight in the body to enable perfect alignment

~The hips and the shoulders are always aligned

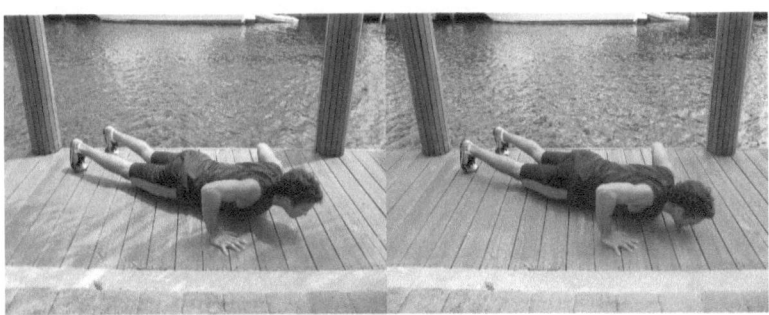

~SLOWLY LOWER YOUR BODY WITH ABSOLUTE CONTROL AND THEN PAUSE

~LOWER YOUR BODY FLAT AGAINST THE FLOOR, ENSURING ALIGNMENT

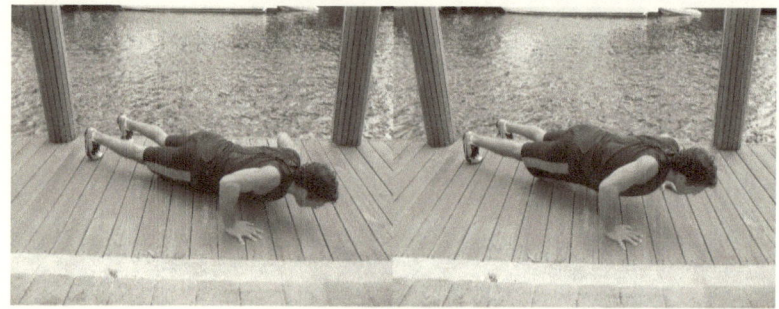

~BREATH OUT WHEN YOU PUSH YOUR BODY UP, EXTENDING YOUR ARMS

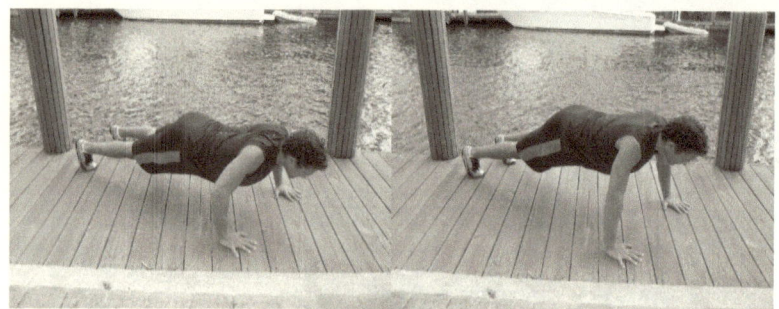

~FULL EXTENTION TO GET A PEAK FLEX OF THE TRICEPS; ARMS STRAIGHT

~REPEAT UNTIL LACTIC ACID ACCUMULATES

~PUSH YOURSELF UNTIL YOU ARE UNABLE TO ACHIEVE PERFECT FORM

Foundational Pushup

Steel Shirt

A pushup can be performed in thousands of different ways. A pushup can be done with perfect form and yield unconceivable results. A pushup can also be done in a manner that exasperates pain and/or increases dysfunction. A pushup must be taken in steps of progression. A pushup should be practiced to perfection until more than 20 repetitions can be performed with ease and in perfect form. When you can do 20 repetitions in perfect form, a progressive exercise should be added to your exercise program. A pushup alternative may be to place your hands on a higher surface, with your feet remaining on the floor. A simple progression is to lower your platform -placing your hands on a lower surface- to decrease resistance. Moving your hands from a kitchen table to a lower coffee table can provide a small increase in resistance.

The foundational pushup should be modified to your fitness level. This can be done without any specific equipment, even if the bare floor is your gym. By placing your hands on a higher level, such as a table or chair, you will decrease the resistance of the pushup. This modification will put more (beneficial) stress on the abdominals as compared to a pushup on the ground with bent legs (on your knees instead of your feet). Alignment must be taken into account as with all of the body's joints. Your elbow should be directly over your wrist, and your shoulder should be directly above your elbow. When you lower your body down with absolute control, place the center of your chest (at the nipple) directly between your two hands. Imagine a string tied to your thumbs, and the center of your chest touches that string at the bottom of the motion. If you did this pushup on a higher surface (like a table) as a modification, the center of your chest (at the nipple) would gently be lowered to touch the table.

You must progress in your intensity or you will not progress in your fitness level. You must change your workouts, order of exercises, repetitions, sets, and exercises on a regular basis. It will make your workouts more exciting and productive. Your workouts will remain efficient enough to provide a challenging anaerobic activity in just one minute.

Improving upper body strength will increase blood flow helping with ailments from arthritis to neuropathy (symptoms include the feeling of pins and needles in the extremities). The importance of dexterity within the hands cannot be underestimated. Your hands are in use every day. The movement of your shoulder is called upon every day. Shoulder injuries can be crippling and cause expensive, time-robbing surgery and physical therapy. All the muscles in your shoulders, wrists, hands, chest, and stabilizing muscles in your abdominals and surrounding your spine will be strengthened and protected from injury with the proper use of this single exercise.

33 repetitions in a minute will make you healthier

YOGA SQUAT – HEELS~UP SQUAT

~FEET SHOULDER WIDTH APART; KNEES AND TOES POINT FORWARD

~LOWER YOUR BODY WITH ENOUGH CONTROL TO STOP AT ANY TIME

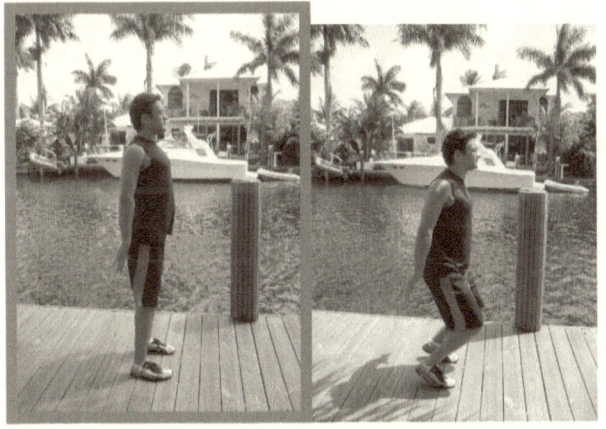

~LOWER YOUR BODY LIKE A SPRING, AND GENERATE ENERGY

~SLOWLY BEND YOUR KNEES

~SQUAT UNTIL YOUR HAMSTRINGS TOUCH YOUR CALVES

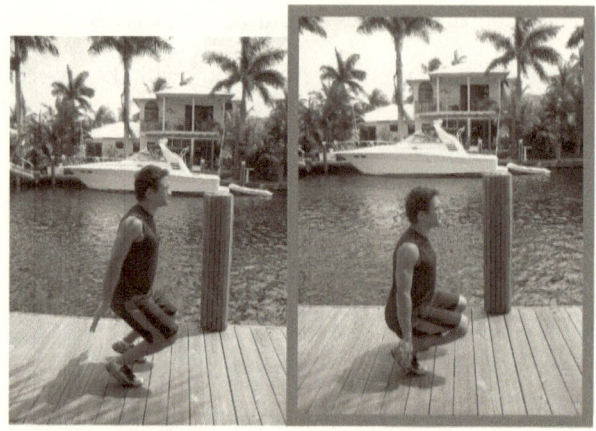

-Breathe all air out on the way down

-Lower your body slowly and pause at the bottom

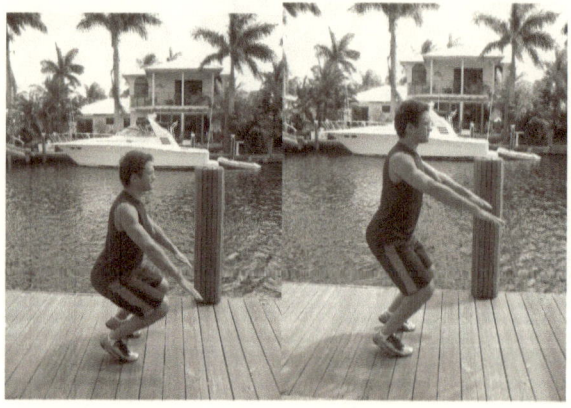

-Pain-free range of motion until you can touch the ground

-Fill your chest with air (until it gets bigger) from the diaphragm

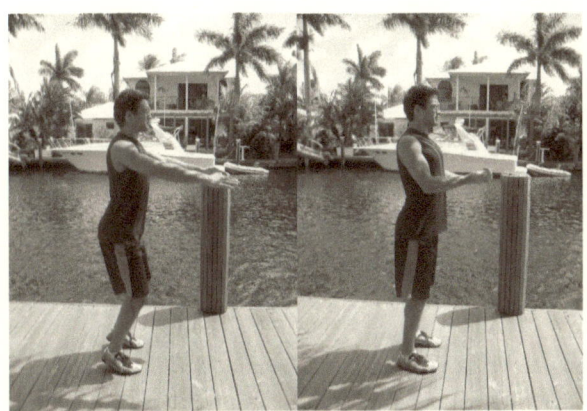

~LOWER BACK FLEXED AND ABDOMINALS TIGHT SO SHOULDERS ARE OVER HIPS

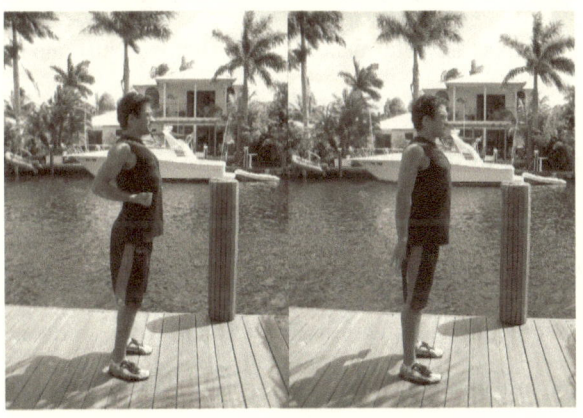

~DRIVE YOUR BODY UP WITH PERFECT POSTURE

~MAINTAIN YOUR SHOULDERS ROLLED BACK, DIRECTLY OVER HIPS

Yoga Squat

Heels-up Squat

This single exercise can bring you unlimited health. It will demand cardiovascular health by instantly putting you in an anaerobic threshold. Your heart rate will be so high that you will be out of breath and technically, you will be in oxygen dept. This will increase your metabolism for hours in just one minute, repeating this exercise 30 times. In less than three minutes, you can do 100 Yoga or Hindu squats that will not only maintain your good health and fitness level but will increase your fitness level. Most people cannot do 100 Yoga squats with no rest. If you perform 100 Yoga squats throughout the day in sets of 10 (every day), you will be able to do 100 non-stop repetitions within 30 days. If you cannot do one Hindu squat, have no fear, you are lucky you have more progress to look forward to than most! There are many alternatives that will prepare you for a Yoga squat, such as doing the exercise in a doorway using your arms to stabilize you. Start with a small range of motion that is pain-free and increase your range of motion every time you practice.

There should be no pain during any exercise. You should not feel this exercise in your knees. You should feel contractions and eventually a burning sensation (lactic acid) in the muscles *surrounding* your knees. Your quadriceps, hamstrings, and gluteus maximus are the main large muscles involved in this exercise. If performed correctly, this exercise will work every muscle in your body. Your body should be tightly flexed with perfect posture. Your shoulders should be rolled back so that they are aligned perfectly over your hips throughout the range of motion.

The range of motion should be perfectly controlled, as you lower your body like a spring, you will generate energy. Pause at the bottom of the exercise, continuing to build up energy like a coiling spring. Maintain your balance and pause at the bottom, touching your hamstring to your calf, while maintaining perfect posture (shoulders aligned over hips). Rise up with an ever so controlled driving force (buttocks muscles) until you are upright with perfect posture, as if standing in a military camp line.

There should be absolutely no rest at the top of this motion. Repeat another repetition of the exercise immediately. As soon as your legs are completely extended and your heels touch the ground, you will go down into another squat. Your legs are straight only for a fraction of a second. The pace is generally two seconds on the way down and one second on the way up, although your speed will increase over time and with practice. You will find a comfortable speed in which you should hear no cracks in your knees, no pain, no problem with balance, and enough speed (without momentum) to get a great workout in just one minute. In just five minutes, you will be challenged enough to create micro-tears in your muscle and permanently increase your metabolism by building functional lean muscle tissue.

Proof of this is being sore the next few days. Micro-tears in the muscle heal overnight (and may take up to 72 hours to heal), and muscle then is built. **When muscle goes up, body fat goes down, metabolism goes up, and the body will appear leaner because, pound for pound, muscle tissue is much smaller than body fat.** Muscle also protects the body, acting as a shock absorber to your joints, ligaments, tendons, and collagen.

25 repetitions in a minute will make you healthier

YOGA PUSH UP

~FEET ABOUT 1 ½ SHOULDER LENGTHS APART

~HIPS AS HIGH AS POSSIBLE

~BACK STRAIGHT AS IF A STEEL ROD REPLACED YOUR SPINE

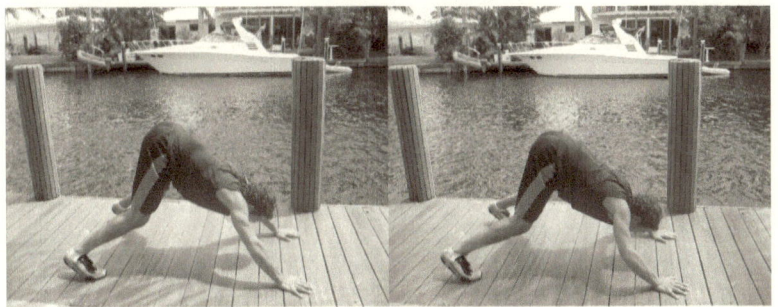

~HANDS AS CLOSE TO FEET AS POSSIBLE, KEEPING YOUR SPINE STRAIGHT

~BEND YOUR ARMS IN THE DOWNWARD MOTION

~YOUR FACE AND CHEST BRUSH AGAINST THE GROUND

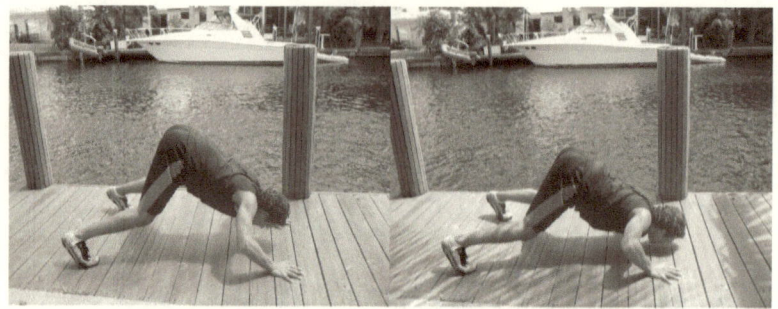

~Keep arms straight until you're able to bend elbows as in picture

~With a slow and controlled motion, dive toward the ground

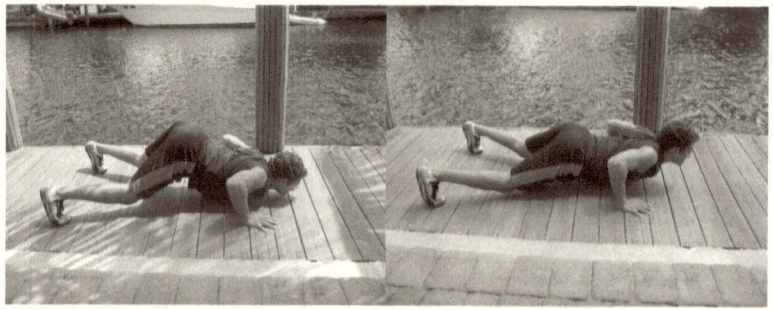

~Control the muscles surrounding the spine and abdominals

~Hold the finish position for ½ second

~Position hold should be similar to upward dog in yoga

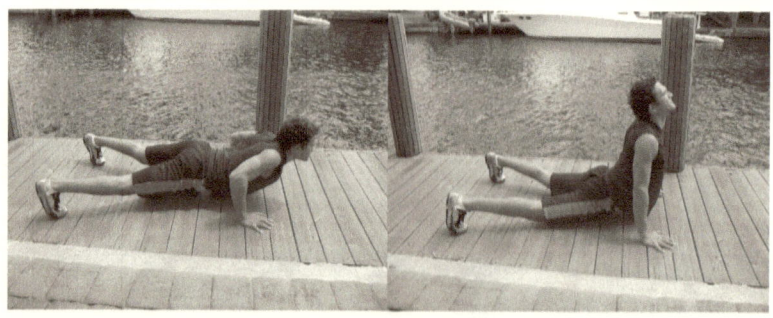

~LEGS HOVER ABOVE GROUND, NOT IN CONTACT

~SHOULDERS ROLLED BACK, LOOK UP WHEN IN FINISH POSITION

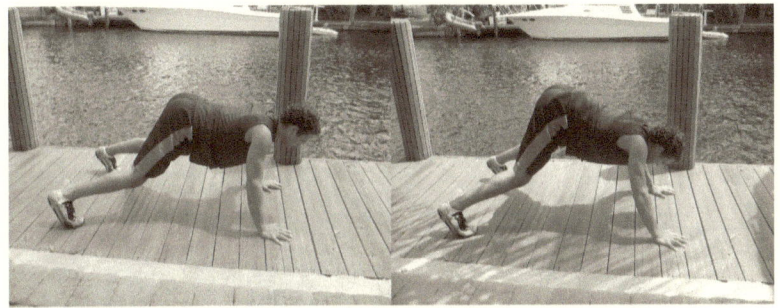

~PULL THE HIPS UP FORCEFULLY TO THE START POSITION

~POSITION HOLD SHOULD BE SIMILAR TO DOWNWARD DOG

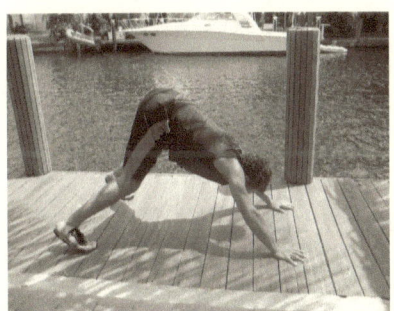

~BREATH IN DEEPLY AS YOUR HIPS PULL UP TO START POSITION

~BREATH OUT AS YOU START OVER

Yoga Pushup

Yoga pushup is an exercise that has unlimited benefits. It can increase flexibility throughout the body, especially in the spine where flexibility is often limited and needed. Lack of flexibility can limit your strength and cause frequent pain from tight muscles. A Yoga or Hindu pushup can improve your range of motion and shoulder health, including the rotator cuff. This exercise is not just for flexibility it will provide incredible strength gains.

The range of motion of a Yoga pushup can never be duplicated on a machine or with free weights. It will work the chest throughout a plane of motion that is almost impossible to adapt to. If an exercise is difficult to adapt to, then the potential for increasing your fitness level is greatly increased. Not only will Yoga pushup increase strength, but it will increase power due to the need for speed and control within this exercise.

To start this exercise, you must have your feet about one and a half shoulder lengths apart. Your feet should be a good bit wider than your shoulders so you can stay stable and increase flexibility. Keep your eyes focused behind you, looking between your legs. Optimally, you will focus your eyes between your hands. If a string were attached to your thumbs, you would stare at the center of that string. Your back is perfectly straight as if a steel rod is your spinal column. The first motion is a controlled swoop, as if you are diving into a pool of water. **Keep your eyes focused on the path that your body is traveling, mimicking the swooping motion that resembles diving into a pool and coming up for water (similar to a dolphin jumping in and out of the water).** It is essential to pause at the bottom when in upward dog (looking up with hips to the ground and shoulders up). Your hips and legs hover just over the ground as you are looking forward with shoulders rolled back. This should somewhat resemble the Yoga position upward dog. Both the start and finish positions should be held for a minimum of a half of a second. **The hold in the start and finish positions should be perfect in form and stability, guiding the motion of the exercise.**

33 repetitions in a minute will make you healthier

PLEA SQUAT

~POINT TOES OUTWARD AND POINT KNEES OUTWARD

~PLACE FEET WITH YOUR HEELS SIX INCHES APART

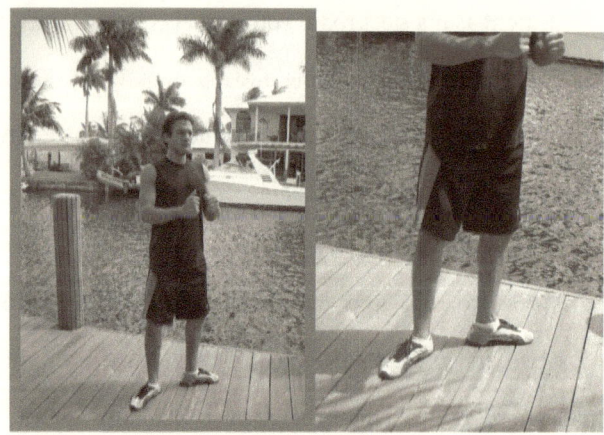

~SLOWLY LOWER YOURSELF WITH COMPLETE CONTROL

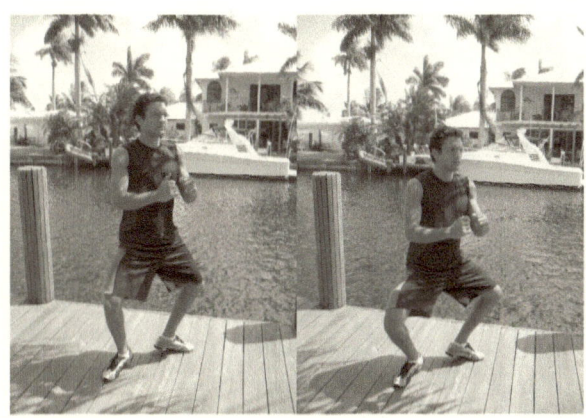

~Raise your heels as high as possible as you lower your body

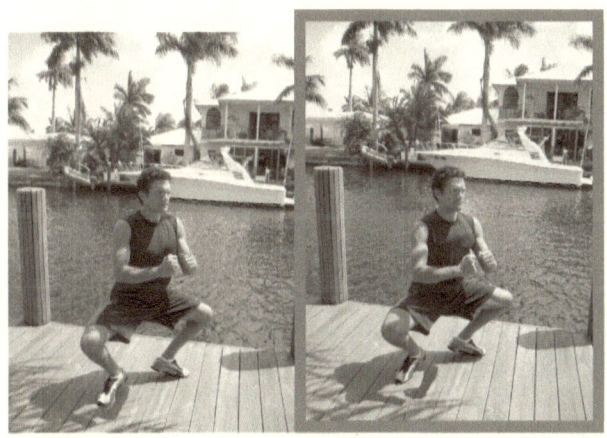

~Keep your shoulders perfectly over your hips

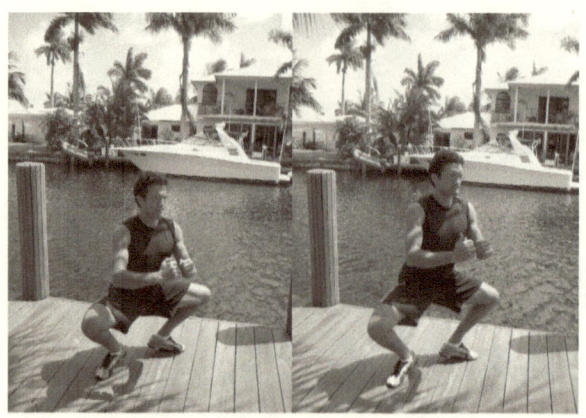

~KEEP ABDOMINALS AND LOWER BACK MUSCLES TIGHT AND FLEXED

~KEEP BUTTOCKS, CALVES, AND ALL OF YOUR LEG MUSCLES AS TIGHT AS POSSIBLE

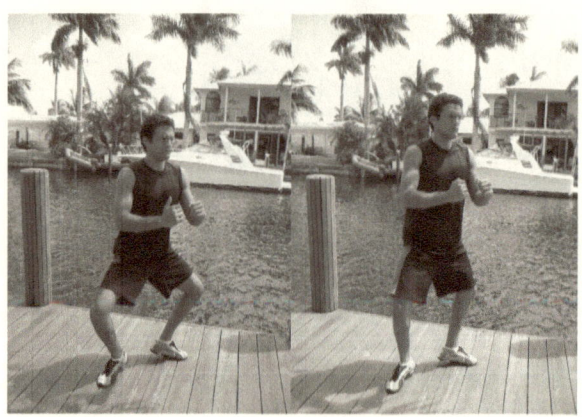

~KEEP HANDS IN FRONT OF BODY AND ARMS BENT TO ASSIST BALANCE

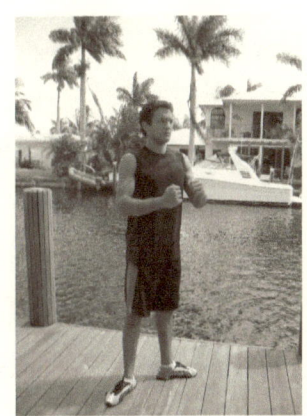

~PERFECT THIS MOTION AND INCREASE REPETITIONS

Plea Squat

Of course this exercise can save your life! The plea is a great alternative to other squats due to the ease of the motion. It is a very natural motion, following the anatomy of your hips, as it allows for your knees and toes to point outward. This may be more pleasing to the knees when a prior condition or injury exists. Although the plea is an exercise you will feel more comfortable performing, that does not mean it is easy. When performing exercises you will attain comfort after time, when form is captured to perfection. You must perfect the form of the motion until there are no flaws. This can easily take a lifetime.

Your feet should be a little closer together than shoulder width apart. Point our toes and knees outward about 90 degrees. Your heels will rise as you lower your body. As your knees bend, completely control your body to prevent momentum and bounce, which can cause stress on the knees (with little-to-no added benefit). Maintain perfect posture; keep your shoulders directly over your hips, which is more easily attained in the plea than other squats. **Imagine your hips and shoulders are the four corners of an unbendable board** (this should be imagined for virtually every exercise except abdominal exercises). Pausing at the bottom of the exercise will prevent momentum. Tighten your abdominal and lower back muscles, while keeping control after the pause, as you extend (straighten) your legs until upright.

The plea should become rhythmic (no bouncing) with no rest or exaggerated pause at the top of the motion. Begin the exercise with your hands in front of your body with elbows bent. Let your hands move freely in a circular motion, if desired, to increase balance and mental readiness. **Exercise is 90% mental and 10% physical.** Push past the burning sensation (lactic acid) localized to the muscle, and maintain absolutely perfect form. You will demand physical fitness and health from your body. You will increase blood flow, increasing the productivity in your life by the boost of motivation that follows a healthier lifestyle. It is as simple as one minute of practicing your plea. Increase your activity over time to progress toward a five minute workout, and you be astounded with the results you will achieve in just minutes a day...the time it takes to brush your teeth!

30 repetitions in a minute will make you healthier

ELBOWS~IN PUSHUP

~Plank position with wrists in line with lowest rib

~Weight focused on the palms of the hands, fingers stabilized

~Abdominals, buttocks, and muscles surrounding armpits TIGHT

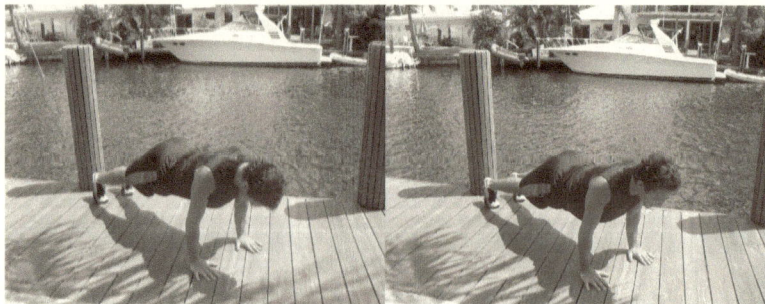

~Slowly lower your body with absolute control

~Tuck your elbows in until they make contact with your body

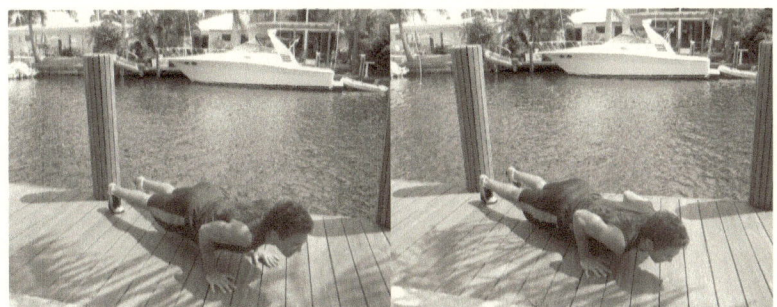

~LOWER YOUR BODY FLAT AGAINST THE FLOOR ENSURING ALIGNMENT

~TIGHTEN MUSCLES IN THE BODY TO ENABLE PERFECT ALIGNMENT

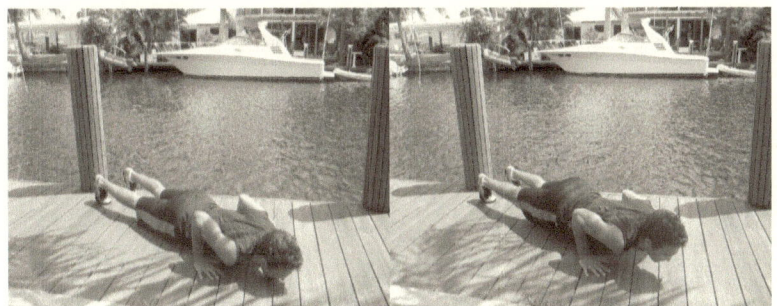

~THE HIPS AND THE SHOULDERS ARE ALWAYS ALIGNED

~THE SPINE IS IMAGINED AS A STEEL ROD, PREVENTING RISK OF INJURY

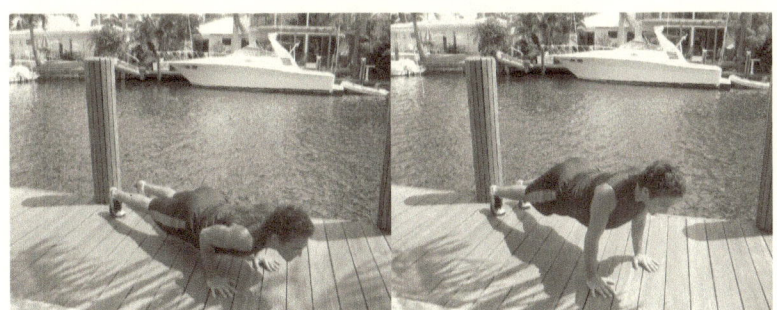

-Breath out when you push your body up, extending your arms

-Fully extend your arms to get a (peak) flex of the triceps

ELBOWS~IN PUSHUP

Keeping your elbows tucked (compared with the foundational pushup) in will put added (and beneficial) stress on your triceps, lower back muscles, and abdominal muscles. This will greatly benefit your body as it will further increase your fitness level, progressing from a foundational pushup. This pushup has alternatives, as does the foundational pushup. You can progress from a traditional pushup, to a modified pushup with elbows tucked in. Progressing from a foundational pushup to an elbows-in pushup may be too difficult. The exercise must be done in perfect form or the modification must be performed until the progression is made to allow for perfect form.

The modified pushup is a great alternative when perfect form cannot be achieved. There are two options for a modified pushup. If a table or bar is available you can decrease the resistance by placing your hands on the elevated platform and your feet on the ground. The center of your chest should touch the platform. If there was a string attached to your thumbs, the center of your chest would touch the center of this string. This cue is very important to obtain perfect form. Your shoulders should be directly above your wrists. Your body should be stiff and straight; image that your hips and shoulders are the four corners of a board. This same form should be exemplified when doing either pushup, modified or not. When a platform is not available, you can bend your knees, changing the leverage. Your knees will be on the ground instead of your feet, but your body is still perfectly straight. Allow your body to go all the way down to the ground to "feel" what muscles are tight when in perfect form− stay straight throughout the motion.

Intensity should always be monitored by lactic acid. You should generally perform as many repetitions as you can until you feel a burning sensation in the localized muscle that you are exercising. Start with five to 10 repetitions and perfect form. You may progress by practicing the exercise every day, or a minimum of three times a week. If you feel very sore in that muscle, then rest that specific muscle one or two days. There have been studies about muscle healing more effectively when an exercise is performed, so do not become sedentary for even one day. Doing 50 to 100 pushups in perfect form consecutively can be a challenging goal that will assist in losing weight and becoming healthier, including cardiovascular heart health. Heart health is greatly increased when there is no rest in your workout as it will challenge your heart and cause physical adaptation.

60 repetitions in a minute will make you healthier

ABDOMINAL CRUNCH

~LIE ON YOUR BACK WITH YOUR SHOULDERS ON THE GROUND

~TUCK YOUR HEAD THROUGHOUT THE MOTION

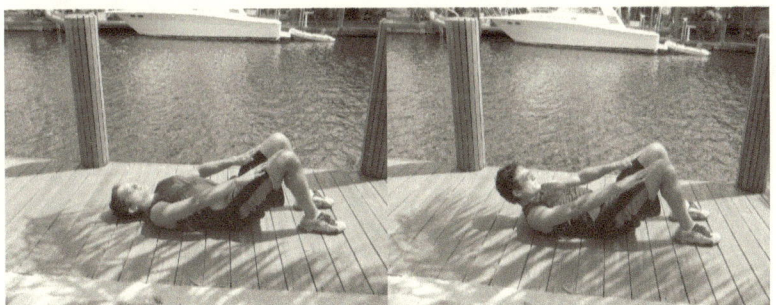

~IMAGINE YOU ARE HOLDING A RACQUETBALL UNDER YOUR CHIN

~STRAIGHTEN YOUR ARMS AND PLACE YOUR HANDS ON YOUR QUADRICEPS

~WITH CONTROL, LIFT ONLY YOUR SHOULDER BLADES OFF THE GROUND

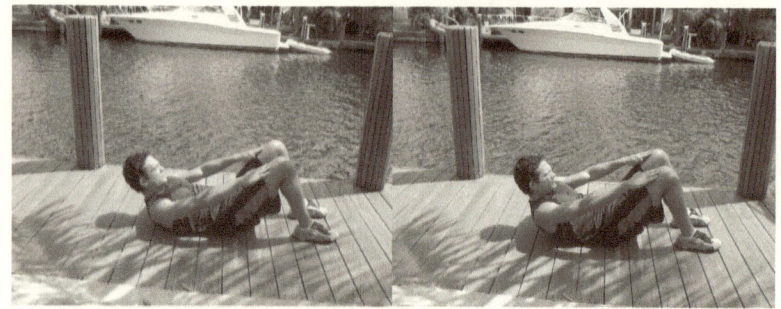

~KEEP YOUR ARMS STRAIGHT THROUGHOUT THE MOTION

~TOUCH YOUR KNEES AND HOLD POSITION

~EXTENDED PAUSE AT THE TOP

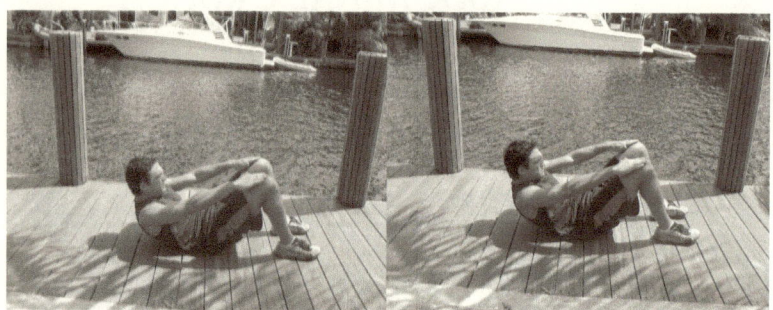

~SHOULDER BLADES ARE NOT IN CONTACT WITH THE GROUND

~YOUR NECK MUSCLES SHOULD NOT REST

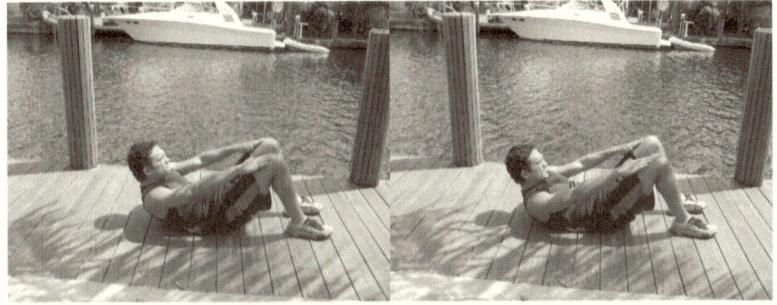

~YOUR HEAD MUST REMAIN TUCKED DURING THE ENTIRE EXERCISE

~LOWER YOUR BODY UNTIL YOUR SHOULDER BLADES REST ON THE GROUND

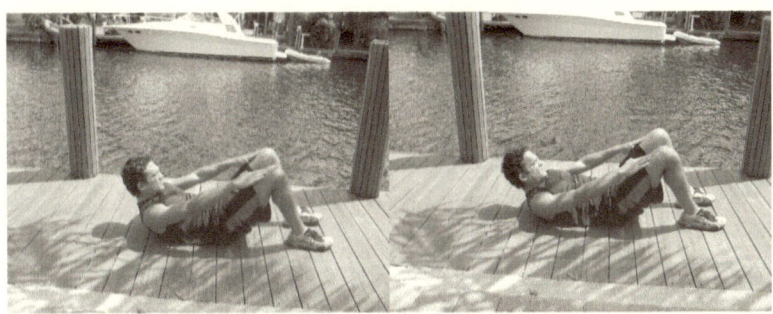

~REPEAT UNTIL LACTIC ACID ACCUMULATES, UNTIL IT BURNS

~STOP IF THERE IS PAIN—PAIN IS AN INDICATION TO STOP

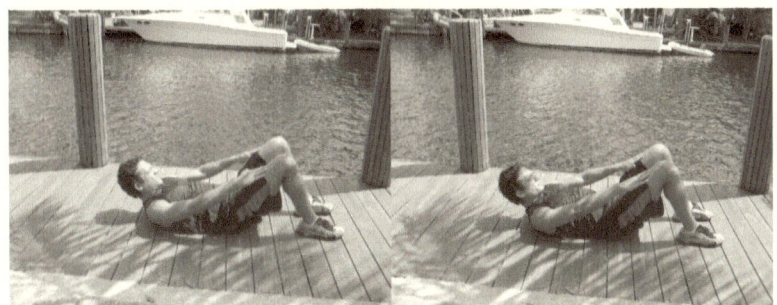

ABDOMINAL CRUNCH

Abdominal strength has nothing to do with the appearance of a six-pack or a flat stomach. Practicing abdominal exercises has relatively nothing to do with reducing abdominal fat. Repeating abdominal exercises will tear down abdominal muscles. Micro-tears in your muscle then heal overnight while you sleep. If you are sore after a workout this is proof of the micro-tears in your muscle. It takes 48 to 72 hours for a muscle to heal. The muscle will heal, which will increase metabolism and reduce chances of injury-but will not reduce or burn body fat in a certain area-spot reducing is impossible.

Abdominal exercises need not be done daily. They should be of the least importance regarding your training. Abdominal exercises should be more thought of as an active recovery, an exercise done in between more difficult exercises to maintain movement and an elevated heart rate. Abdominal exercises do not burn many calories, and do not increase your metabolism as much as the exercises that use larger muscles. Foundational squats and foundational pushups burn more calories, and increase your metabolism more dramatically than any abdominal exercise. You may contract your abdominals more doing a squat or pushup compared with abdominal exercises, according to various published studies. Body fat will leave your body in the same order that it first accumulated. It will most likely leave your stomach last. A flat stomach or six-pack is dependent upon your body fat percentage. Doing hundreds of crunches or sit-ups will not get you a six-pack unless you burn thousands of calories to create a calorie deficit or increase metabolism.

Doing abdominal exercises will help develop abdominal muscles to assist your body in more complex movements, using larger muscle groups. Abdominal muscles will be used in every exercise if you are doing the exercises properly.

Maintaining good posture with your shoulders over your hips demands abdominal muscle recruitment. Lower back muscles are the antagonistic muscle group to your abdominals. The lower back (lumbar spinae) is flexed during every exercise if it is performed properly. The "core" muscles are activated during all exercise, the epicenter of the body–the abdominals and lower back muscles. It is not necessary to perform isolation exercises for the abdominals, because the "core" muscles are worked in every exercise when done properly. If you increase the contraction (flex your muscles) of your core muscles, you will improve your posture immediately.

The importance of abdominal exercises should not be exaggerated. If you overdo abdominal exercises, you will over-train, and neglect the efficient and more effective exercises that will decrease the size of your belly. Overtraining interrupts the healing of the muscle. Abdominal exercises do very little to decrease the size of your stomach. The focus of your exercise program should be performing exercises that work large muscle groups, like the foundational squat and pushup. Evolving to more difficult exercises is of much more importance than increasing the difficulty of abdominal exercises.

The abdominal exercises shown in this book are intended for active recovery or "cool-down cardio" to keep your heart rate up, offering absolutely no rest during your workouts. Make your workouts short and sweet. No need for rest.

The foundational crunch is a small movement. Lie on your back with your arms straight, and place your hands on your quadriceps. Keep your arms straight; do not bend your elbows. Keep your chin tucked as if you are holding a blue rubber racquetball under your chin. If you are having trouble with keeping your chin tucked, or have pain in your neck, then actually hold a ball under your chin. The motion is very small. Your fingertips touch your knees as your shoulders will leave the ground– pause–and slowly lower your body back to the lying flat position. Only your shoulders should leave the ground while the rest of your back is stabilized and firmly planted on the ground. This movement is referred to as spinal flexion. This is one of the very few exercises in which you will bend your back. As you apply the slight bend in your back, your abdominals will tighten and contract. Continue this movement with no rest until lactic acid forms, and the burning sensation stops your movement.

30 repetitions in a minute will make you healthier

REVERSE CRUNCH

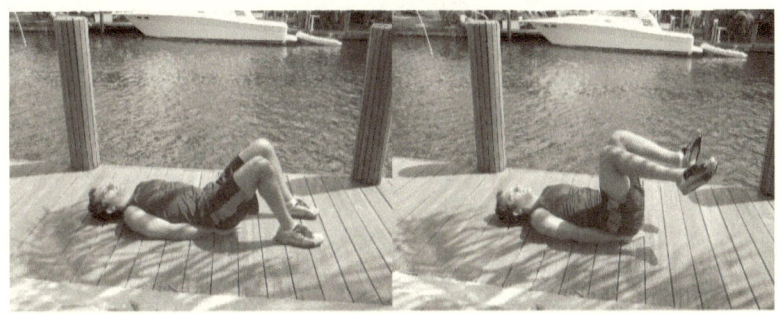

~PLACE YOUR HANDS UNDER YOUR TAILBONE OR HIPS

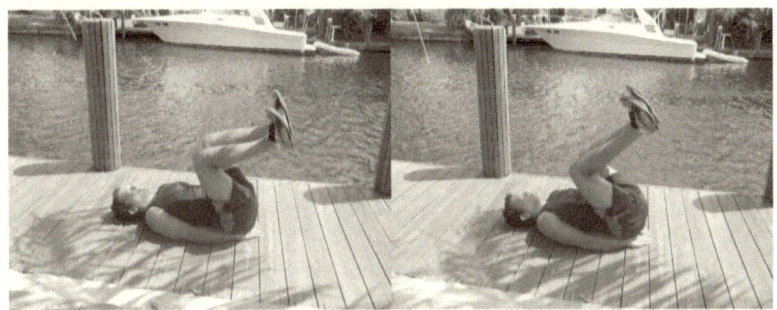

~KEEP YOUR HEAD, NECK, AND SHOULDERS ON THE GROUND

~KEEP YOUR NECK RELAXED IN CONTACT WITH GROUND THROUGHOUT MOTION

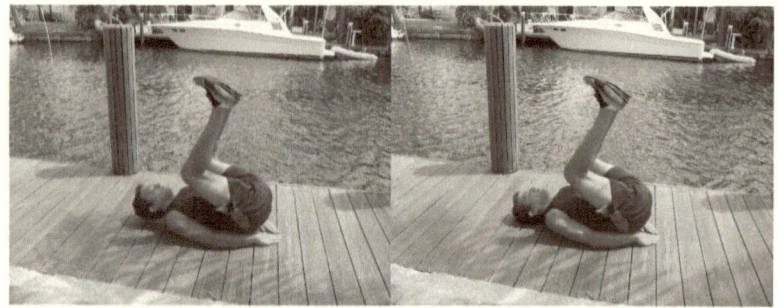

~A FORCEFULL CONTROLLED MOTION SHOULD LIFT YOU

~SLOWLY LIFT YOUR HIPS, LOW BACK AND MID~BACK OFF THE GROUND

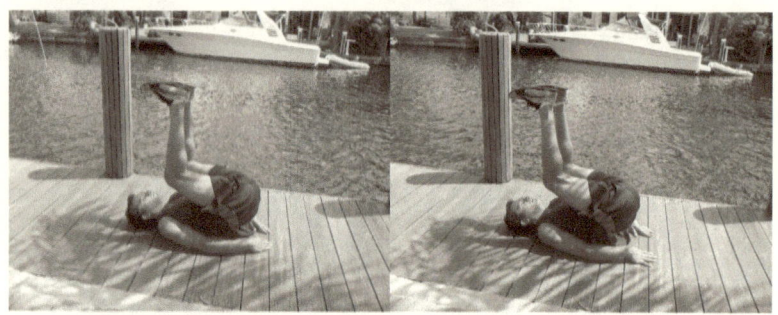

~PAUSE AT THE TOP OF THE MOTION FOR ½ SECOND

~SEPARATE THE UP AND DOWN MOTION WITH THIS POSITION PAUSE

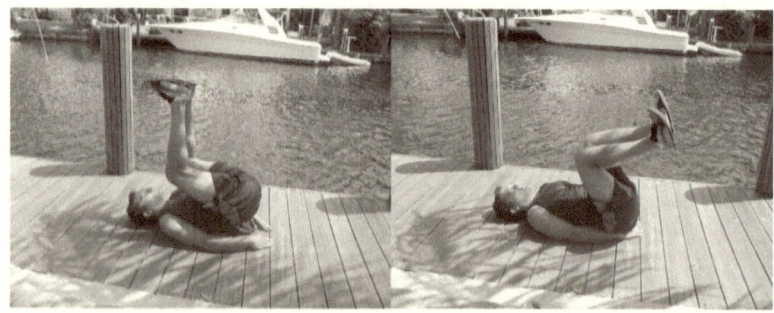

~ROLL BACK TO THE START POSITION

~ROLL BACK WITH A MOTION TWICE AS SLOW AS THE ROLL UP

~KEEP A 90° BEND IN YOUR LEGS THROUGHOUT THE MOTION

REVERSE CRUNCH

The reverse crunch is an abdominal exercise that targets the "lower abs." In reality, the contraction of your abdominal wall is "all or none." The abdominals that make up the "six-pack" are your abdominal rectus. In a reverse crunch, the abdominal contraction begins with the lower abdominals, and then the upper abdominals are contracted. Your abdominals are a very important muscle group, as they are worked in every exercise if done properly. Always remember that the appearance of a six-pack or flat stomach is based on body fat percentage (total body fat), not abdominal strength.

The reverse crunch should be done with absolute control. First, lie on your back and give yourself plenty of support by placing your hands underneath your tailbone or next to your hips. When you roll back, you might want to adjust your hand position to apply more stability. Your head, neck, and shoulders should rest on the ground throughout the exercise. Force and power are applied as you roll back lifting your hips, lower back, and middle back off the ground. There should be no pain or pressure on the neck. This should NOT be a "jump" or a jerky motion– the force used is highly controlled. Lift your hips off the ground, and then increase your range of motion over time, as you progress to the optimal range of motion. Hold a controlled pause at the top of the motion. When rolling down to the start position, you should be extremely controlled with the ability to stop your range of motion at any time within the exercise. **Stopping the motion in EVERY exercise at ANY time is an essential component of form.** The roll back to start motion should be twice as slow as the initial forceful roll back to shoulders position.

Just as with every exercise, there should be absolutely no pain. Shorten your range of motion until there is no pain and you can progress pain-free. An exercise must be excluded from your workout program until your body is strong enough to perform the exercise pain-free. The exercises in this book will allow your body to progress until they are all perfect, but this is not an overnight journey. If you stay dedicated for just one to five minutes daily you will get results. Try dedicating the length of time it took for your body to create an unhealthy state– when ignoring healthy eating and exercise. Just one to five minutes daily. If you skip one day, you should double up! If you dedicate just one minute to exercise and skip one day you have to exercise for two minutes the next day, four minutes the day after, and eight minutes if you miss three days. Dedicate yourself to a healthy, happy, fit, and better-looking body–just one-minute minimum every day!

40 repetitions (on each side) in a minute will make you healthier

TRANSVERSE CRUNCH

~LIE ON BACK WITH SHOULDERS ON THE GROUND

~TUCK YOUR HEAD THROUGHOUT MOTION

~IMAGINE YOU ARE HOLDING A RACQUETBALL UNDER YOUR CHIN

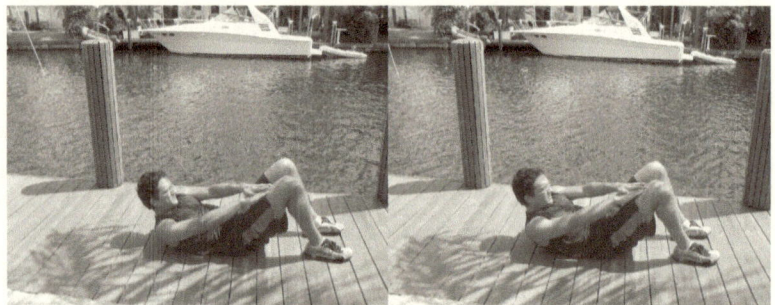

~STRAIGHTEN YOUR ARMS AND PLACE BOTH HANDS ON ONE LEG

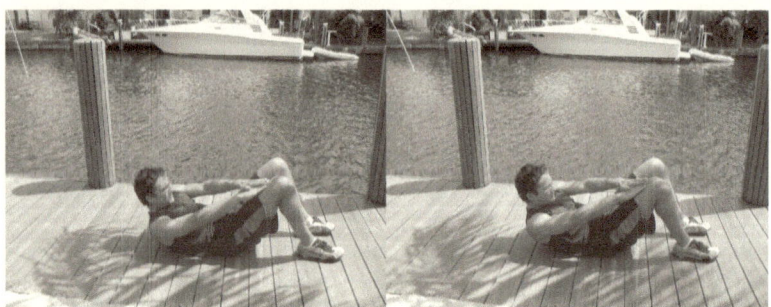

~SLOWLY, AND CONTROLLED, LIFT ONLY ONE SHOULDER BLADE

~LIFT YOUR SHOULDER UNTIL IT IS OFF THE GROUND

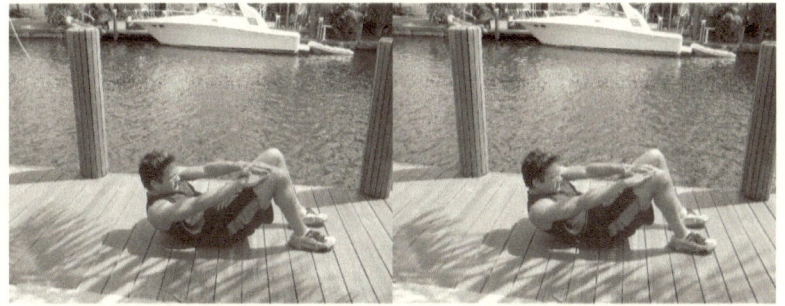

~Keep your arms straight throughout the motion

~Touch your knee and hold position to separate the motion

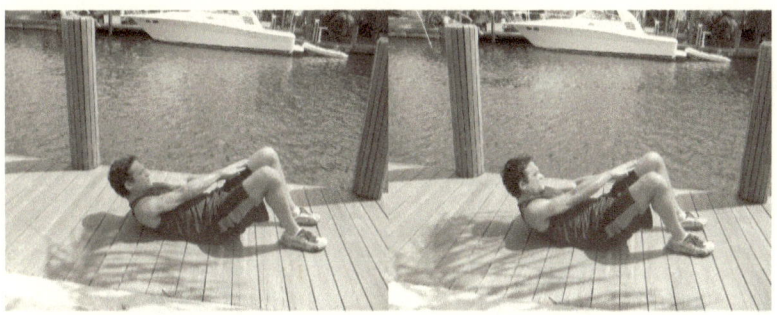

~Repeat this exercise on the same side

~Repeat until it burns and then switch sides

~Pause at the top when your shoulder blade is off the ground

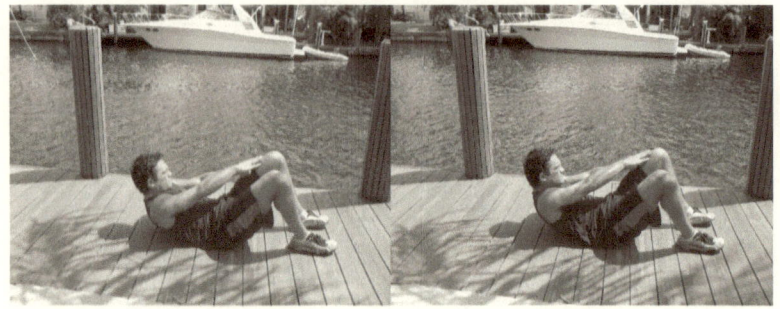

~SLOWLY LOWER YOUR BODY UNTIL YOUR SHOULDER BLADE IS BACK ON THE GROUND

~YOUR NECK MUSCLES SHOULD NOT REST

~YOUR HEAD WILL REMAIN TUCKED DURING THE ENTIRE EXERCISE

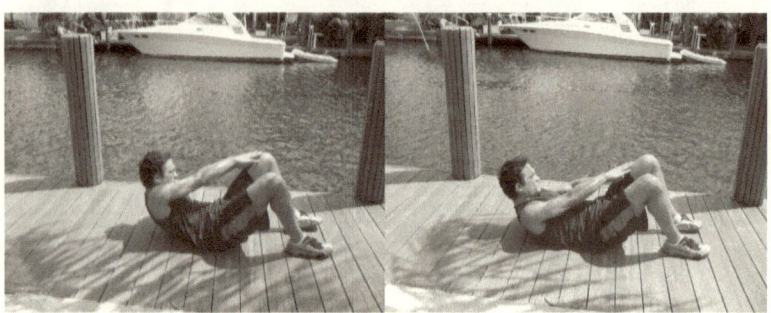

~MAKE CONTACT WITH YOUR KNEE

~BOTH FINGERTIPS OF THE MIDDLE FINGER SHOULD TOUCH THE KNEE

TRANSVERSE CRUNCH

Abdominal exercises should not be your primary exercises. These exercises are in this book to act as an active recovery. The exercises that work larger muscle groups are far more valuable, efficient, and effective. The transverse crunch is very similar to the abdominal crunch. It is performed crossing over with your hand on only one leg. This will activate another muscle in the abdominal cage. The muscle is the transverse abdominals. If you made an X over your belly button it would diagram your transverse abdominals. The transverse crunch will also work the abdominal rectus.

Perform this exercise repetitively on one side until lactic acid accumulates and you feel a burning sensation in the muscle. As you repeat the exercise, your shoulder blade should touch the ground after every repetition. Your head should remain tucked as if you are holding a blue rubber racquetball (or something comparable in size larger than a Ping Pong ball and smaller than a tennis ball) under your chin throughout the movement. Your head should touch the ground only before and after you have completed an entire set of repetitions. If your neck is not stabilized as if you are holding a ball under your neck, it will hurt. Stop and correct the motion. Your neck should be just about the same distance from your chin as it would be if you were standing in perfect posture. Your neck should not be pulled back like a turtle, and your chin should not be glued to your neck. Your chin should not move close to your body and then far away from your body as if you are nodding yes to a question.

40 repetitions in a minute will make you healthier

BACK EXTENSION

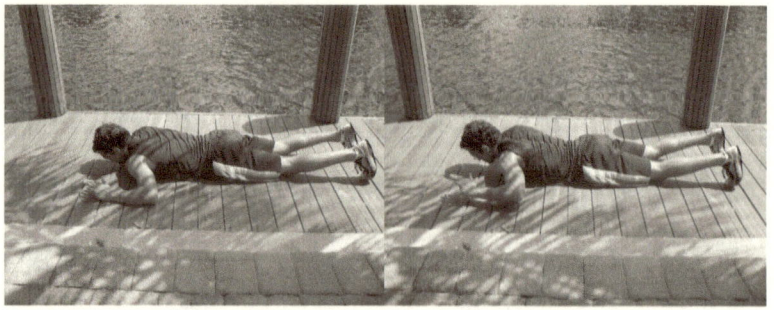

~LIE ON STOMACH AND KEEP THIGHS AND TOES ON THE GROUND

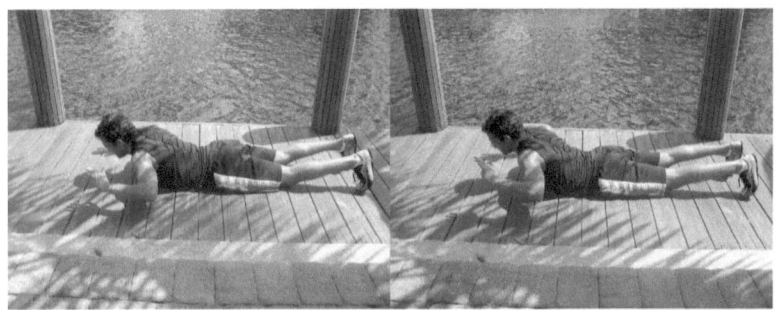

~SLOWLY, AND CONTROLLED, LIFT YOUR CHEST OFF THE GROUND

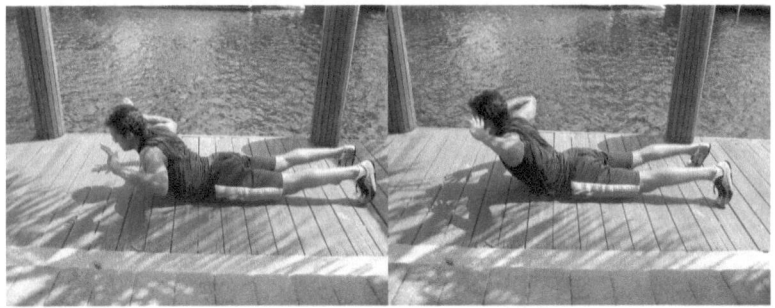

~LIFT YOUR CHEST AS HIGH OFF THE GROUND AS POSSIBLE AND PAUSE

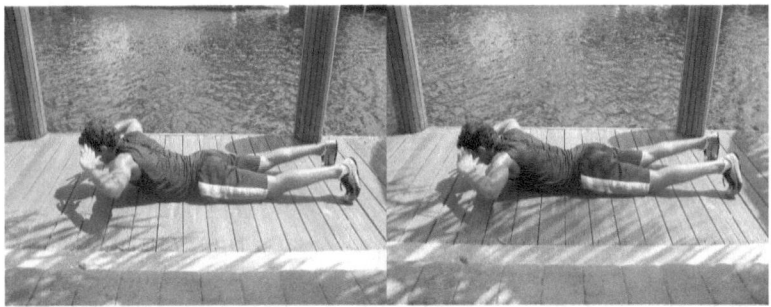

~SLOWLY LOWER YOUR BODY TO START POSITION

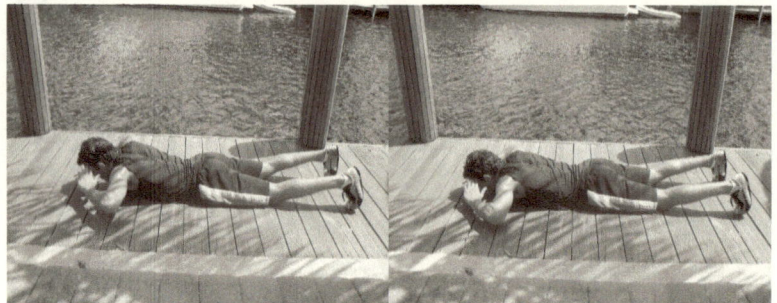

-Your chin shoud be able to touch the ground in the end postion

Back Extension

Lower back strength is essential for a pain-free life. The plexus of nerves surrounding the lower back can distribute pain throughout the body. The center of the nervous system surrounds the spine. Strengthening the muscles surrounding the spine strengthens the entire body. The muscles surrounding your spine will protect your nervous system, and eliminate pain, acting as your personal chiropractor.

The lower back muscles, lumbar spinae, are used in every exercise to stabilize– similar to the constant utilization of abdominal muscles. Because the lower back muscles are always in use it is not necessary focus on them.

Lower back exercises such as the back extension should not be overused. The lower back extension can be used as an active recovery just like abdominal exercises. The back extension does not burn as many calories as the squats and pushups that are described in this book. The back extension will not burn a lot of calories or make a large impact on metabolism. It is very useful to strengthen your back muscles, improve posture, and alleviate pain.

You must know why you are doing each and every exercise. Without a reason there is no purpose, and no truth or belief in the exercise. The words that fill this book are more than just words–they are truths and that is why Organic Fitness works, and why I believe in it.

Lie down on the ground or a bench with your chest facing the floor. Place your hands about one to three inches above your shoulders. With a slow and controlled movement, lift your chest off the ground. Use your hands to stabilize this movement by pressing your fingertips to the ground (helping your lower back) to lift your chest off the ground. Progress and strengthen your lower back muscles until you can lift your chest off the ground with your hands in the air or in slight contact with your head. Your lower back is the primary muscle lifting your body. Keep your legs and thighs on the ground. Pause at the top of this motion with your chest off the ground for at least half a second, and then slowly lower your chest back to the ground.

After practicing this exercise, you will not need the support of your hands on the ground, and you will be able to keep your arms bent with your fingertips barely touching your head. Repeat this exercise until you feel a slight burning in the muscle (lactic acid), but be careful to not injure the delicate lower back by overdoing this exercise. Progress slowly. Even if you do only five perfect repetitions for the first week and then increase to 10 repetitions for another week, by the third week you will be able to perform 15 repetitions.

Epilogue

Organic Fitness will work if you dedicate yourself with a

positive attitude. Only one minute a day can make an immaculate change

and keep you healthy. If you dedicate five minutes a day doing these

exercises that can be performed anywhere you will be healthy. You will

prevent death from mortality, and protect your body from sickness while

you are alive. As little as one to five minutes a day will change your life.

Be creative; combine these 10 exercises to make innumerable workouts.

Focus on one muscle group one day, and total body the next day. Or

practice just one exercise, another the next day, and then alternate

between the two on the third day. Do not constantly work a sore muscle; if

a muscle is sore then work a different muscle for a day or two. Let's keep it

simple for now. Stay active with these 10 exercises until they are perfect

in form.

I developed Organic Fitness after more than 10 years of helping people

achieve their goals. Regardless of age, gender, or injuries, I guarantee

results–getting to your goal–when you follow my program. I spend more

than 10 years researching health and fitness and studying the

physiological aspects of health promotions. I earned a master's in nutrition

from the University of Bridgeport, and a bachelors of science in exercise

and health sciences at Kennesaw State University. I witnessed thousands

upon thousands waste their time in corporate, community, and commercial fitness centers and gyms. In the time it takes to get to a gym, you can achieve the best workout of your life–anywhere. These are God's movements–sitting and standing, pushing yourself up from the ground. Being able to run, jump, love, and play ARE God's movements. Enjoy these movements, embrace these workouts, breathe deep, and love life.

Keith J. Lopez, M.S., B.S.

TheOrganicWorkout.com

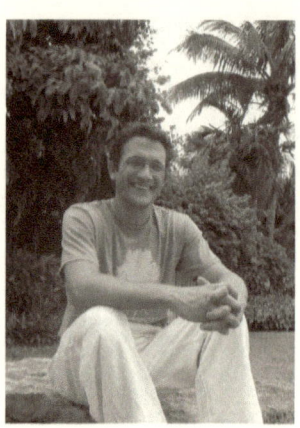